The Hypothyroid Menu:
Eating Well With The Natural Approach To Hypothyroidism

I0434950

Table of Contents

Introduction

I want to thank you and congratulate you for downloading the book, *"The Hypothyroid Menu: Eating Well with the Natural Approach to Hypothyroidism."*

This book explains what hypothyroidism is, what its causes are, and how it is treated. It discusses some natural methods to manage hypothyroidism and help people avoid having this disorder.

This book further enumerates foods that should be included in the diet of a person with hypothyroidism, as well as foods that should be avoided. Finally, sample recipes are provided to give readers an idea of what a "hypothyroid-friendly diet" is like.

Thanks again for downloading this book, I hope you enjoy it!

Chapter 1: What Is Hypothyroidism?

Are you tired all the time? Are you gaining weight even though you don't overeat? Do you have brittle nails and dry skin? If you notice these things happening and you don't know why, it could be that you have an underactive thyroid gland. A lot of women have this condition, especially older women, although it remains undiagnosed for most of them. Some men have it too, as do children and babies.

The medical term for an underactive thyroid gland is hypothyroidism ("hypo" is a prefix meaning "low" or "below normal"). It is estimated that about 2% of women and less than 0.5% of men in the United States have hypothyroidism. Babies and children can have it too, but it is more common among women aged 60 years and above. Up to one-tenth of all women in this age range have symptoms of this disease.

In hypothyroidism, the problem is an impaired thyroid gland that does not produce enough thyroid hormone. This affects how energy is processed and utilized by the body.

Let's take a closer look at the root of this illness: the thyroid gland. This is a butterfly-shaped gland found in the lower front part of the neck, just below the Adam's apple in men. It is the largest of all endocrine glands in the body. Like other glands, the thyroid gland secretes hormones. The main hormones it produces are called thyroxin (T4) and triiodothyronine (T3), or simply thyroid hormones.

As these hormones circulate through the bloodstream, they affect the whole body, including vital organs such as the heart and the brain and large areas like the skin and muscles. The greatest impact of the hormones is on the body's metabolism.

Hypothyroidism slows down metabolism, the body's built-in mechanism to produce and utilize energy.

With insufficient thyroid hormones, the body makes less energy, which explains why a person with this condition gets tired very easily. His body also has a harder time burning down calories, which is why he tends to gain weight quickly. The simple fact is that a sluggish metabolism affects practically all the processes that take place in our body. Heart rate, breathing, digestion, temperature regulation, mental processes and growth are all adversely affected by a slow metabolism.

The opposite of all this can happen in another health condition called hyperthyroidism ("hyper" means "over" or "above."). Here, there is an overproduction of thyroid hormone, resulting in a faster-than-normal metabolism. Energy is quickly produced and also quickly used by the body; hence the person with hyperthyroidism appears hyperactive and needs to eat often to replenish his energy. But he does not gain weight despite eating a lot. Hypothyroidism is a more common ailment than this reverse condition called hyperthyroidism.

Chapter 2: What Causes Hypothyroidism?

There are many known causes of hypothyroidism. First, it can be inherited from a parent with a defective gene (on chromosome 2) that affects the production of thyroid hormones. Interestingly, people with other genetic abnormalities (such as Down syndrome and Turner's syndrome), may also suffer from hypothyroidism.

A second and more common cause, especially in the United States, is an autoimmune condition called Hashimoto's thyroiditis (or Hashimoto's disease). What happens here is that the body's malfunctioning immune system produces antibodies that attack the tissues of the thyroid gland. This harms the thyroid gland, such that it cannot produce sufficient amounts of thyroid hormone. If Hashimoto's thyroiditis is not treated, the attack can go on until the thyroid gland is eventually completely destroyed.

For some reason, women have a greater susceptibility to Hashimoto's thyroiditis than men. Statistics indicate that the risk factor for this disease among women is up to eight times higher than men's.

Certain medical treatments in the neck area can also cause hypothyroidism. Some people have their thyroid gland wholly or partially removed to cure a hyperthyroid condition; as a result, they can develop hypothyroidism later on. People with cancer who are receiving radiation therapy on the neck region are also prone to hypothyroidism.

Many of the treatments for hyperthyroidism are in fact a potential cause of hypothyroidism. The most drastic of these treatments is, of course, the surgical removal of the thyroid gland. More moderate therapies include radioactive iodine treatment and taking medication that reduces the functioning of the thyroid gland. All these can lead to a hypothyroid condition.

Another cause of hypothyroidism is lack of iodine in one's diet. Iodine is needed by the thyroid gland for it to function properly. When there is a chronic lack of iodine in the diet, the thyroid gland secretes insufficient amounts of hormones. In advanced cases, the gland can noticeably enlarge, and this is called goiter.

Iodine deficiency is not very common in the United States and other first-world countries because iodine is almost always added to salt during manufacturing. It is in underdeveloped countries that iodine deficiency is more prevalent.

Other possible causes of hypothyroidism include:

- Certain medications – A number of drugs can slow down the production of thyroid hormones. Among them are lithium (used to treat bipolar disorder), amiodarone (to treat heart problems), and interferon alpha (for cancer treatment).

- Pregnancy – Some women experience an inflammation of the thyroid after giving birth. This is called "postpartum thyroiditis." It is characterized by an acute increase, then a severe decline, in thyroid hormone levels. The condition often resolves spontaneously after some time.

- Neonatal problems – A few babies are born with congenital hypothyroidism. It could be caused by genetics or by malnutrition of the mother during pregnancy. Newborn infants are routinely screened for hypothyroidism in hospitals.

- An abnormality in the pituitary gland or the hypothalamus – The pituitary gland in our brain secretes a hormone called thyroid-stimulating hormone (TSH). Meanwhile, the hypothalamus produces a hormone called thyroid-releasing hormone (TRH). If either of these hormones is in short supply, due to a malfunctioning pituitary gland or hypothalamus, the thyroid gland also cannot produce enough thyroid hormone. This is called "secondary hypothyroidism" given that the problem isn't the thyroid gland itself but something else. When it is the thyroid gland that is malfunctioning, the condition is referred to as "primary hypothyroidism."

Chapter 3: How To Find Out If You Have Hypothyroidism

There are tell-tale signs that could indicate the presence of a hypothyroid condition. The most common of these signs and symptoms are:

- Chronic fatigue and weakness

- Mental sluggishness, forgetfulness, or the inability to concentrate

- Muscle aches

- Dry, scaly skin

- Hair loss, or dry, coarse hair

- Brittle nails

- Slow speech

- Slow heart rate

- Mood swings, which may include depression and irritability

- Unexplained weight gain (or difficulty losing weight)

- Constipation

- Sensitivity to cold temperatures

- Irregular (heavy) menstrual period

- Swollen thyroid gland (goiter)

The frequency and intensity of these symptoms depend on how long the hypothyroid condition has been there, and the amount of thyroid hormone that is produced by the body. If there is a very pronounced shortage of this hormone, then the symptoms will be more severely felt.

Not all the listed symptoms are likely to be experienced by a person with hypothyroidism. Just a few of these could be present, and they could easily be mistaken for the normal signs of aging. These symptoms could also gradually arise over some time; hence there is a tendency to overlook them.

If you know of someone who is experiencing some of these symptoms, without any apparent explanation for them, then he or she could be suffering from hypothyroidism. The odds increase when the person is female and in her sixties, and when there is a family history of thyroid disorders. The odds are also higher if the person has diabetes or rheumatoid arthritis.

Once hypothyroidism is suspected, the sensible thing to do is to see a doctor and get one's thyroid hormone levels tested. A simple blood test usually suffices for this. Other doctors use more sophisticated tests such as thyroid scans.

With the use of radioactive iodine or other media, these scans provide an accurate picture of the thyroid gland and the parts of it that are not actively producing hormones. Scans also show the presence of lesions, nodules, cysts or any inflammation that could be interfering with thyroid function.

Clinical tests can show the stage at which the hypothyroidism is. There is mild or early-stage hypothyroidism if the T4 levels are lower than normal but not severely so. It is also indicated if the T4 levels are normal, but the TSH levels are above normal. It is important to identify the stage of the disorder so that the doctor can come up with the appropriate treatment plan.

Chapter 4: Conventional Treatment For Hypothyroidism

Once diagnosed, hypothyroidism treatment should commence right away so that the person will no longer experience the symptoms he had which interfered with normal living. If untreated, the symptoms may become worse over time and make life even more difficult.

There could also be serious complications that would be much harder to treat. These include heart problems, infertility, obesity, and a condition called Myxedema. Myxedema is the most serious form of hypothyroidism, and it is life-threatening. A person with Myxedema can suddenly fall down and lose consciousness, experience seizures, slip into a coma, become hypothermic (have a very low body temperature), and die.

Of course, several factors are considered when deciding which mode of treatment is most appropriate for a patient suffering from hypothyroidism. The factors that are taken into account are: how long the disease has been there, the actual thyroid hormone levels (how much they deviate from normal values), the severity of the symptoms experienced, and the physical condition of the patient.

For mild, early-stage forms of the disease, simple treatment plans often suffice. The doctor prescribes thyroid hormone pills, which are synthetic equivalents of the hormone T4. These should be taken orally daily, exactly according to the doctor's orders. The medication usually takes effect within a few days, and the person notices an easing of the symptoms he had. Within a few months, the symptoms often disappear completely.

Even so, the pills still have to be taken daily, for as long as one lives. Periodic follow-up visits to the doctor are necessary to monitor hormone levels and see if an increase or a decrease in the dosage is called for. It usually takes a few dosage adjustments over time before the right dosage is determined— one that allows the correct hormone levels to be reached without any unpleasant side effects. This treatment is called hormone replacement therapy.

Sometimes, all that a doctor prescribes is a change in the person's diet or lifestyle. This happens when the hypothyroidism is very mild and the symptoms experienced are minor. But the patient is advised to keep an eye on his symptoms and report any change. If the symptoms worsen, a more serious treatment plan may be warranted.

In the case of secondary hypothyroidism, in which the cause of the disease is not the thyroid gland itself but some other organ in the body (such as the pituitary gland or the hypothalamus), the underlying cause should be treated. The appropriate course of treatment is determined by a physician after a series of consultations.

Likewise, when hypothyroidism is caused by the autoimmune disorder called Hashimoto's thyroiditis, then this underlying condition should be addressed. Some doctors believe that nine of out of every ten people with hypothyroidism have Hashimoto's. This implies that many hypothyroidism sufferers should consult a professional about how to treat Hashimoto's as well if they have it. Attacking the root cause of the hypothyroidism makes more sense than simply ingesting pills to treat the symptoms.

Chapter 5: Natural Means To Treat Hypothyroidism

There are certain natural means that anyone can use to help maintain the health of his thyroid gland and avoid hypothyroidism. These methods also help in preventing further deterioration of the thyroid gland if some impairment has already started and it has begun to secrete lower-than-normal levels of thyroid hormone. These natural methods work best in the early stages of the hypothyroid disorder. More advanced stages of the disease will need conventional treatment, often through hormone replacement therapy.

The first natural means to treat hypothyroidism is adopting a thyroid-friendly diet. This is a diet consisting of foods rich in iodine, protein, healthy fats, vitamin D, selenium and iron. Good protein sources are nuts, legumes and organic eggs.

Soy and soy-based products should be avoided, including tofu and soy milk. Non-starchy vegetables (rather than grain-based ones) are also good for thyroid health. Good sources of healthy fats are olive oil, avocados, nuts, fish, coconut milk products, and yogurt. (These recommended food choices for healthy thyroid function will be discussed in greater detail in the next chapter.)

Apart from diet, another natural method to avoid hypothyroidism or to manage it is by engaging in activities that raise one's metabolism. As discussed earlier in this book, the major effect of hypothyroidism is slowing down the body's metabolic functioning. Here are some ways to reverse this effect and keep our metabolism up and running:

- Exercise regularly. Exercise and physical activity keep the metabolism up and running. Being sedentary slows down metabolism.

- Build up your muscles. Lifting weights at the gym (or elsewhere) will help one to develop lean muscle mass. This will boost the metabolism, even when the person is at rest and doing nothing.

- Drink water often.

- Get enough sleep at night. Lack of sleep and irregular sleeping hours can wreak havoc on your metabolic function. Make sure you get six to nine hours of good sleep each night.

- Don't eat heavy meals. It is better to eat small and more frequent meals rather than indulging in the traditional three (or two) heavy meals every day.

- Don't skip breakfast. At the very start of the day, rouse your metabolism by taking a light, protein-rich breakfast.

- Don't rely too much on so-called metabolism boosters such as hot peppers, green tea, and caffeine. Studies have shown that they increase metabolism only by a negligible amount and temporarily.

Apart from exercising and eating right, one should also practice relaxation and stress management. The thyroid is one of the most sensitive and reactive glands in the endocrine system. Under heavy stress, the thyroid gland could go into distress mode and fail to function properly.

Exercises

Consult your doctor before you start any exercise program and discuss its benefits and ask for his suggestions for the best exercises for you.

Choosing the right exercise can help you overcome the symptoms of hypothyroidism. Initially start exercises slowly. Increase it day by day. You should exercise for at least 45 minutes to an hour.

Low impact aerobic exercises at least 5 times a week is helpful. With low impact aerobics, your heart rate increases and it does not put too much pressure on your joints.

A recumbent bike or a stationary bike is very helpful for cardio exercises. You can go cycling outdoors too.

Walking is a good exercise too.

To increase the metabolism goes in for strength training.

There are some very good exercises which are good for hypothyroidism.

Learn the correct techniques from a qualified trainer.

Exercises: Some of the exercises are which suitable for hypothyroidism are:

- One legged dead lift
- Overhead press
- Squats
- Push ups
- Rowing on a rowing machine etc.

Yoga and Meditation: Treat hypothyroidism in a natural way through yoga and meditation. Yoga is a Hindu ancient spiritual method where certain body postures, meditation and breathing exercises are practiced. It helps bring a balance of the mind and body. Yoga originated from India. It can be practiced by people of any age groups.

Learn the proper yoga techniques from a qualified yoga trainer.

Practicing yoga on a regular basis will help you. People have claimed to be happier, less stressed and in general a feeling of well being since they have started practicing yoga. Yoga and meditation helps you reduce stress to a very great extent. The different postures are called **asanas**. The breathing exercises are called **pranayam.** The meditation is called **dhyan.**

The following Asanas are known to be helpful in hypothyroidism:

- Sarvangasan also known as shoulder stand
- Matsyasana also known as Fish pose
- Marjariasan also know as cat pose
- Halasan also known as plough pose
- Janu shirasana also known as one legged forward bend
- Viparitakarani also known as inverted pose
- Surya namaskar also known as sun salutation
- Bhujanasana also known as cobra pose
- Paschimottanasan also known sitting forward bend
- Naukasan also known as rowing pose
- Pavanmuktasana also known as wind relieving pose
- There are many more asanas

Pranayam: There are many different breathing exercises called pranayam. They are very useful for those suffering from hypothyroidism. Pranayam are known to give energy to the body. Pranayam increases blood circulation in the body. It relaxes and soothes the nerves and body in general. You will feel more active. It increases the oxygen intake in the body. The following pranayam are known to be helpful in hypothyroidism.

- Kapalbhatti (skull shining breathing technique) - kapal means forehead and bhati means shining
- Anulom vilom - Alternate nostril breathing
- Ujjayi pranyam (also called as victorious breath or ocean breath technique) is highly recommended for hypothyroidism
- Suryabhedan pranayam with kumbhak – breathing with right nostril only and kumbhak means retaining of breath after deep inhalation
- Bhastrika pranayam with kumbhak – called bellows breathe also.
- Bhramari pranayam – bumble bee breathing

Meditation helps relieve stress. It is a way of life. It means to put an end to thought process. Meditation is to reduce the activity of the mind. Try to keep your mind free of thoughts.

Chapter 6: What To Eat To Prevent And Treat Hypothyroidism

Eating well becomes much more important when one is suffering from a disorder such as hypothyroidism. There are certain foods to avoid, and other foods to consume more of. If the person with a hypothyroid condition isn't conscious about what he eats, he could inflict more harm to his thyroid gland and see a worsening of the symptoms of the disease.

What makes matters worse is that with hypothyroidism, the person feels tired and weak most of the time and his thinking becomes sluggish, so there is a great temptation for him to mindlessly reach for foods that have stimulants and high-sugar content, just so he can "wake up" and be energized. While definitely enticing, these kinds of foods are exactly what he should avoid. Apart from upsetting his blood sugar levels, they can also harm the thyroid gland.

Let's list down the foods that should be avoided by a person who has hypothyroidism.

- High-sugar and high-caffeine foods. These include pastries and all things sweet, and coffee and tea. They are not only unhealthy for the thyroid gland, but unhealthy for the whole body in general. Additionally, some teas (like black and green tea) also contain fluoride, which, according to some studies, weakens thyroid function.

  Speaking of coffee, those who are taking hormone replacement therapy should avoid drinking coffee within an hour of taking hypothyroidism pills. Coffee inhibits the absorption of the medicine, rendering it less effective. The same is true with orange juice. Avoid drinking it close to the time you take your pills.

- Goitrogens – These can inhibit iodine absorption and good thyroid functioning. They include soybeans, kale, broccoli, peaches, Brussels sprouts, peanuts, turnips, cabbage, spinach, rutabaga, cauliflower, kohlrabi, millet, strawberries, watercress and radishes. You may still eat goitrogens, but eat them cooked (never raw) and in moderation. The cooking process usually destroys substances in them that are harmful to thyroid tissue.

- Gluten-rich foods. Gluten and thyroid tissue are very alike in molecular composition. For persons who have Hashimoto's thyroiditis, eating gluten results in an increase in the autoimmune attack on the thyroid gland.

- Any food that the person is sensitive to. Anything that rouses the inflammatory response or tends to cause allergies should be avoided because this disrupts the immune functioning of the body. In the presence of Hashimoto's thyroiditis, this will result in more antibodies attacking the thyroid gland.

Meanwhile, here's a list of food and nutrients that are hypothyroid-friendly. These should be what your diet consists of if you have an underactive thyroid gland:

- Protein – This nutrient is not only essential to our body; it also assists in the transport of thyroid hormones to various cells and tissues. Good protein sources include quinoa, grass-fed meats, legumes, nuts, nut butters, organic eggs, and fish. Remember, however, that soy products, while rich in protein, are not good for thyroid function. Avoid tofu, soy milk, energy bars, and fake "vegetarian" meats. They can disrupt the normal functioning of various hormones in the body.

- Healthy fats – Not eating enough fats and cholesterol could lead to hormonal imbalances. This is because fat is necessary in the transport and absorption of most hormones. Some good sources of healthy fats are ghee, avocados, fish, nuts, nut butters, cottage cheese, yogurt, olive oil, coconut milk products, and flax seeds.

- Glutathione – This is a strong antioxidant that boosts and regulates the immune system as well as heals thyroid tissue. It is highly recommended especially for those who have Hashimoto's thyroiditis. Good sources of glutathione include raw eggs, broccoli, grapefruit, asparagus, avocado, squash and garlic. Other sources are cauliflower and cabbage, which are goitrogens, hence these should be eaten cooked and in moderation.

- Certain vitamins and minerals, including Vitamins A, D, B-complex, iron, zinc, copper, iodine, selenium, and omega-3 fatty acids. These nutrients do not strengthen thyroid function per se, but not having enough of them could aggravate the symptoms of hypothyroidism. Nuts, whole grains, shellfish, dairy (whole wheat bread), winter squash and eggs are good sources of these nutrients.

- Tyrosine – This is an amino acid (protein) that helps promote mental alertness and reduce depression. It has also been found to soothe the skin by preventing dryness and wrinkles. Tyrosine can be found in wheat, beans, oats, fish, nuts, eggs, meats and dairy products.

Probiotics – These are supplements that promote good digestion by ensuring there is a good amount of healthy bacteria in the intestinal tracts. Thyroid function is aided by the presence of these healthy bacteria.

Nutrition In Hypothyroid Diet

In hypothyroidism, the body cannot prepare its own iodine. With a few dietary alterations, you can help yourself to fight the problem better. The diet for a person with hypothyroidism should contain foods rich in iodine and vitamins like Vitamin C, E, Vitamin B2, B6, riboflavin, zinc etc. They provide nutrients for proper functioning of the thyroid as well as good health in general.

The different necessary nutrients are:

- Poultry food like eggs, chicken, turkey, duck
- Seaweed like kelp
- Sea food like tuna, salmon, shrimp, cod, crabs, oysters etc.
- Milk products like cow's milk, yogurt, goat's cheese etc.
- Nuts like almonds, Brazil nuts, peanuts, macadamia nuts, hazelnuts etc.
- Vegetables like asparagus, onions, garlic, ginger, chilli, potatoes, sweet potatoes, bell peppers, egg plant, mushrooms, beetroots, carrots, cucumber, tomatoes, zucchini , leeks, black and red radish etc.
- Herbs like parsley, cilantro, rosemary, mint, Siberian ginseng, etc.

- Sunflower seeds
- Meat like fresh pork, lamb, beefs etc.
- Whole food like brown rice, different types of beans, chickpeas etc.
- Fruits like Pomegranates, apples, grapes, mangoes, pineapples, oranges, kiwis, bananas, avocados, plums, cantaloupe, grape fruit, papaya etc.
- Berries like blueberries, cranberries, blackberries, raspberries etc.
- Oils like extra virgin olive oil, coconut oil, fish oil etc.
- Cooked red cabbage and broccoli not more than twice a week
- Evening primrose oil
- Apple cider vinegar
- Guggul – consult your doctor before having this

Hypothyroidism is a lifelong problem. You can manage it with diet and exercise. Eat a healthy diet. Your priority should be to take care of yourself. Set realistic goals, try to lose weight. The best way to keep in check with hypothyroidism is control your diet and stress and do exercise.

1. Change your life style: Eat a healthy diet, incorporate exercises in your daily routine. Be positive. Try to achieve your goal.

2. Change your diet: Reduce your carbohydrate intake. Go in for complex carbohydrates like fresh fruits, vegetables, whole grains etc.

- Reduce simple sugars like in cakes, cookies, ice creams etc.
- Drink at least 8 glasses of water every day.
- Increase your fiber intake.

3. Exercise: Hypothyroidism generally causes weight gain. Exercise is very necessary to lose weight and in general to reduce the feeling of fatigue. You might feel very tired very quickly but do not give up. Keep trying, you will succeed one day.

4. Reduce your stress: Stress increases hunger. Reduce your stress. It goes a long way. For this deep breathing exercises   are   very   helpful.

Chapter 7: Thyroid-Friendly Recipes

In this chapter are three simple recipes that work great for people with hypothyroidism, as well as those who wish to prevent having this disorder.

It's good to remember that eating five to six small meals in a day is preferred to taking larger, fewer meals. This helps to keep the metabolism at a steady rate, avoiding surges and dips in energy levels. It also aids in weight loss. Thus, simple and easy-to-prepare meals are best, and the recipes below are good examples.

Blackberry Smoothie

This can be a snack at anytime of the day, or a breakfast food to get your day started in an upbeat mood. It too can be a workout drink. It contains lots of protein, good fats, and fiber. Although low in sugar, a glassful is enough to make you feel satisfied and nourished.

Ingredients:

- Organic blueberries - about a handful
- Hemp seeds - as much as desired
- Almonds, walnuts or pecans – a handful
- Ghee (or coconut oil) - 1/2 tsp
- Milk whistle - 1 tbsp
- Ground flax seed - 1.5 tbsp
- Camu Camu powder - 1/2 tsp
- Warm water – 1 cup
- Raw honey - 1 tsp

Preparation:

1. Place all ingredients in a blender.
2. Blend until desired consistency is reached.

Note that a number of hypothyroid-friendly foods are found in this recipe. Ghee, hemp seeds, almonds, blueberries, and flax seeds are especially good for people with an underactive thyroid gland. While sweet-tasting and energizing, this drink is low in sugar, making it an ideal choice.

Beet Roesti with Eggs, Asparagus and Ham

Ingredients:

- Asparagus – 1 bunch
- Beets – 3 large pieces
- Fresh rosemary – 3 sprigs
- Rice or spelt flour – 1/3 cup
- Vegetable oil
- Butter
- Iodized salt
- Poached eggs – optional, as desired
- Slices of ham – optional, as desired
- Sour cream (optional)
- Chives (optional)

Preparation:

1. For the pan-roasted asparagus, get the asparagus, butter and salt ready. Melt butter in a frying pan over medium heat.
2. Sautee asparagus until tender. Add salt and butter for flavor as desired.

For the beet Roesti:

1. Peel and shred the beets using a grater or a food processor. Add the chopped rosemary, followed by salt and rice or spelt flour. Combine well.
2. In another, bigger frying pan, heat oil. Add beet mix in pancake sizes; make sure there is enough room to flip.
3. If needed, lower heat to avoid overcooking. After about five minutes, or when you see that a crust has formed at the bottom, flip.
4. Cook until the other side is done. Transfer to a plate.

5. An optional ingredient is pan-fried ham. Slice ham thinly and pan fry in butter until done.

Another optional ingredient is poached eggs. Boil water, and then add a little vinegar. Add the eggs to the boiling water and poach to the desired doneness.

Plate the pancakes, and then add the ham and the eggs. Finally, top with sour cream and chive.

Again, this is a recipe that has foods recommended for persons with hypothyroidism. Asparagus, eggs and iodized salt are excellent choices, and the recipe is very easy to prepare. Even kids will enjoy this recipe as a tasty, nutritious snack or meal.

Fried Egg and Avocado Salad

This is a recipe that makes two servings. Its main ingredients are avocado (rich in good fats and vitamins) and eggs (rich is protein). It is also fiber-rich, helping to ease or avoid constipation which some persons with hypothyroidism suffer from. This recipe can be ready within minutes. It is a light dish that can be eaten as a snack anytime of the day.

Ingredients:

- 1/2 to 1 avocado, sliced
- 4 eggs
- 6-8 leaves, Romaine lettuce
- Sliced almonds
- Butter
- Salt and pepper to taste
- Chives (optional)

Directions:

1. In a pan, melt butter over medium heat. Add eggs and fry to desired doneness.
2. Next, wash and tear lettuce into desired sizes. Place the avocado and almonds on top of the lettuce, then add the fried eggs.
3. Chop chives or scallions; then sprinkle these over the eggs. Finally, season with salt and pepper

Asparagus Soup:

Ingredients:

- 5 ounce asparagus, sliced
- 5 ounce snap peas, stringed, chopped
- 5 ounce fennel bulbs, chopped
- 1 small bunch green onions, chopped
- 2 cups water
- ¾ teaspoon sea salt or to taste
- Pepper powder to taste
- 1 ½ tablespoon brown rice
- 1 large leek
- 1 tablespoon olive oil
- ¼ cup fresh dill
- ¼ cup fresh mint leaves
- 1 ½ cups vegetable broth or chicken broth
- 1 ½ - 2 tablespoons lemon juice or to taste
- Zest of 1 lemon
- Garnish with fruity green olive oil

Method:

1. Wash and slice all the vegetables.
2. Place the asparagus, snap peas and fennel bulbs in a large pot. Add water. Add salt and rice to it.
3. Place the pot over low heat, cover and simmer the vegetables for about ½ an hour.
4. Meanwhile, in a sauté pan heat olive oil, add the green onions, sauté. Add a pinch of salt. Sauté until golden brown. Transfer this to the pot.
5. Add dill, mint and the vegetable broth to the pot. Simmer for a little while more. Remove from heat. Cool.

6. When cooled, blend it in a blender until smooth. Pour it back into the pot.
7. Simmer again. Add pepper powder and lemon juice. Adjust the pepper powder, salt and lemon juice to suit your taste.
8. Pour the soup into soup bowls and put a few drops of fruity green olive oil and serve hot.

Vegetable Soup:

Ingredients:

- 1 small onion, finely chopped
- 1 large carrot , grated
- 1 leek, finely chopped
- 2 new potatoes, grated
- ½ can of flageolet beans
- ½ liter vegetable stock
- Sea salt to taste
- Pepper powder to taste
- Chilli flakes to taste
- 1 tablespoon extra virgin olive oil

Method:

1. Pour olive oil in a pot. Keep the pot on medium heat. When the oil is hot, add onions, sauté for around 3-4 minutes until the onions are pink.
2. Add carrots and potatoes and sauté for 5 minutes more. Add leeks. Sauté for a couple of minutes more until the vegetables are cooked.
3. Add the vegetable stock. When it is boiled, remove from heat.
4. When cooled, blend the contents until smooth. Transfer the contents back to the pot. Add the beans. Simmer for a while – about 3-5 minutes. Add the chilli flakes and adjust the salt and pepper to suit your taste. Serve hot.

Goat's Cheese Salad:

Ingredients:

- 1 bunch rocket lettuce (arugula)
- 2 tomatoes, sliced
- ½ packet goats cheese, sliced
- 3-4 tablespoons Pesto sauce

Method:

1. On a baking tray, lay the lettuce leaves.
2. Place the tomatoes on lettuce leaves.
3. Spread the pesto sauce over tomatoes. Place the sliced goat's cheese over the tomatoes.
4. Bake in an oven until the cheese is softened.

Carrot and Beetroot Salad:

Ingredients:

- 2 beetroots, peeled, shredded
- 3 carrots, peeled, shredded
- 3 springs of thyme (fresh or dried)
- 1-2 tablespoons vinegar
- Sea salt to taste
- Pepper to taste.

Method:

1. Add all the ingredients in a bowl and toss.
2. Refrigerate until use.

Zucchini Salad:

Ingredients:

- 1 medium sized zucchini, sliced
- ½ can anchovies or sardines, mashed with a fork
- 2 tablespoons dill, chopped
- 1 tablespoon olive oil
- Juice of ½ a lemon or to taste
- Sea salt to taste

Method:

1. To make the dressing: In a small bowl, add olive oil, lemon juice and salt. Mix well.
2. In a large bowl, add zucchini, anchovies and dill.
3. Pour the dressing over it and toss.
4. Ready to serve.

Avocado salad:

Ingredients:

- 4 avocadoes, mashed
- 2 tomatoes, chopped
- 1 onion, chopped
- 2 cloves garlic, minced
- 2 tablespoons lemon juice or to taste
- 2 tablespoons cilantro, chopped
- Sea salt to taste

Method:

1. Add all the ingredients in a bowl. Toss well
2. To serve, garnish with cilantro.

Cucumber Sesame Salad:

Ingredients:

- 1 medium sized cucumber (1/2 pound)
- ½ tablespoon dark soy sauce
- ½ teaspoon white sesame seeds, toasted
- ½ teaspoon black sesame seeds, toasted
- Red chilli flakes to taste
- Sea salt to taste
- Pepper powder to taste

Method:

1. Peel the cucumber and remove the ends. Use a julienne blade and cut the cucumber lengthwise.
2. Place the cucumbers in a bowl; add soy sauce, sesame oil, chilli flakes, salt, pepper and the toasted sesame seeds. Toss well.
3. Refrigerate.
4. Serve cold.

Chicken and Bean Salad

Ingredients:

- ½ chicken breast (grilled or poached), shredded
- ¼ cup black beans canned, drained
- ¼ cup corn, canned
- ¼ cup fresh tomatoes, diced
- ¼ cup lettuce, chopped
- ¼ cup carrots, chopped

For the dressing:

- 1 tablespoon plain Greek yogurt
- ½ ounce goat cheese, crumbled
- 1 tablespoons cilantro
- ½ lemon juice
- ¼ avocado
- ¼ teaspoon cumin
- 1 tablespoons water

Method:

1. To make the dressing, blend together all the ingredients of the dressing in a food processor.
2. Add all the ingredients of the salad in a bowl. Pour the dressing. Toss well.
3. Ready to serve.

Red/Black Radish Salad:

Ingredients:

- 6 red/black radish, grated
- 2 fresh tomatoes, chopped
- 2 tablespoons cilantro, chopped
- 1 green chilli, chopped
- Sea salt to taste
- 1 tablespoon lemon juice

Method:

1. Mix together all the ingredients. Keep aside for 30 minutes
2. Ready to serve.

Scrambled Eggs:

Ingredients:

- 2 eggs
- 2 teaspoons olive oil
- Sea salt to taste
- Pepper to taste
- 1 medium carrot, shredded
- 1 medium beetroot, shredded
- 1 lettuce leaf, torn
- 1 scallion, sliced
- 1 avocado , mashed

Method:

1. Make scrambled egg using olive oil.
2. Mix together carrot, beetroot, lettuce, scallion and avocado.
3. Top with scrambled egg to serve.

Almond bread:

Ingredients:

- 5 cups almond meal
- 3 teaspoons arrowroot powder
- 2 tablespoons baking powder
- 2 tablespoons honey
- 6 eggs, beaten
- 2 teaspoons sea salt or to taste
- 1 teaspoon apple cider vinegar

Method:

1. In a large bowl, mix together almond meal, baking powder, salt and arrowroot powder.
2. In another bowl, add beaten eggs, vinegar and honey. Mix well.
3. Add the egg mixture into the almond meal mixture. Mix well.
4. Pour into a greased loaf dish.
5. Bake in a preheated oven at 300 degree F for about 45-50 minutes or until done.
6. Slice. Serve with fresh berries or clear soups.

Homemade Breakfast Cereal:

Ingredients:

- 1 tablespoon chia seeds
- 1 tablespoon hemp seeds
- 1 tablespoon flax seeds
- 1 tablespoon pumpkin seeds
- ½ teaspoon vanilla extract
- 1 small pear, sliced
- 1 tablespoon coconut nectar
- Pinch of sea salt
- 1 tablespoon coconut milk
- 1 tablespoon coconut butter (optional)
- 5-6 almonds, slivered
- Hot water

Method:

1. Grind together chia seeds, hemp seeds, flax seeds and pumpkin seeds. Transfer into a bowl.
2. Add vanilla extract and salt. Mix well.
3. Pour hot water and coconut butter over it.
4. Cover and keep aside for 10 minutes.
5. The mixture would have thickened now.
6. Serve with pears and almonds.

Banana Bread:

Ingredients:

- 4 bananas, mashed
- 3 cups brown rice flour
- 2 teaspoons baking powder
- 1 ½ cups brown rice
- 6 egg whites
- 1 cup raisins
- 2/3 cup apple sauce
- 2/3 cup brazil nuts, chopped
- 2 teaspoons cinnamon powder

Method:

1. Mix together rice flour, cinnamon and baking powder.
2. In a bowl add banana, apple sauce, egg whites and vanilla. Mix well.
3. Add the rice flour and baking powder mixture. Mix well.
4. Add the Brazil nuts and raisins. Mix well.
5. Pour the mixture in a greased loaf dish.
6. Bake in a preheated oven at 350 degrees for about 45 minutes or until well baked with cracks appearing on the top and browned well.
7. Slice and serve.

Date bites:

Ingredients:

- 4 ounce dates, de seeded, chopped
- 2 tablespoons honey
- 2 tablespoon pumpkin puree
- ½ tablespoon chia seeds
- ½ teaspoon ginger, ground
- A pinch of nutmeg powder
- A pinch of salt
- ½ cup old fashioned oats
- ½ cup toasted coconut flakes
- ½ cup pumpkin seeds, toasted
- Few drops of stevia (optional to make it sweeter)

Method:

1. Add dates, honey, chia seeds, cinnamon powder, ginger, nutmeg powder, stevia, pumpkin puree and salt into the food processor. Blend until smooth.
2. Transfer into a large bowl. Add oats, coconut flakes and pumpkin seeds. Mix well.
3. Transfer into a lined baking dish. Press well.
4. When cooled, cut into bite sized bars.
5. Can store up to 2 weeks if refrigerated.

Green Smoothie:

Ingredients:

- 5-6 leaves of lettuce (any variety)
- 1 cucumber, peeled, chopped
- ½ cup zucchini
- Few fresh dandelion leaves
- 2 tablespoons cilantro
- 2 tablespoons celery
- 1 green apple, chopped
- ½ cup carrots, chopped
- Stevia drops to taste
- 2 teaspoons coconut oil

Method:

1. You can use any or all of the vegetables mentioned above.
2. Blend together all the ingredients.
3. Adjust the stevia to suit your taste.

Blue berry Smoothie:

Ingredients:

- 1 cup rice milk, unsweetened
- ½ cup blue berries
- Stevia drops to taste

Method:

1. Blend together the blue berries and rice milk.
2. Add stevia drops to taste.
3. Tastes good, chilled.

Detox Shake:

Ingredients:

- ¼ cucumber
- ½ apple
- ½ banana
- Juice of ½ a lemon
- ¼ chilli pepper (optional)
- 1 clove garlic
- Few leaves of mint or cilantro
- ½ glass water

Method:

1. Add all the ingredients in a blender. Blend until smooth.
2. Tastes best when served chilled.

Banana Smoothie

Ingredients:

- 1 banana, sliced
- 1 cup almond milk , unsweetened or cow's milk
- 1 teaspoon maple syrup or a few drops of stevia sweetener
- ½ teaspoon cinnamon powder

Method:

1. Place the banana slices, almond milk maple syrup, and ¼ teaspoon cinnamon in a blender. Blend well until smooth. Pour in glasses.
2. Sprinkle with the remaining cinnamon.
3. Refrigerate. Serve chilled.

Mushroom Burgers

Ingredients:

- 6 large Portobello mushrooms
- 10 cloves garlic, peeled
- 4 tablespoons balsamic vinegar
- ¼ cup extra virgin olive oil
- 1 cup red onions, sliced
- Sea salt to taste (optional)
- Pepper to taste
- 6 burger buns
- 6 lettuce leaves
- 1 large tomato , sliced into 6 pieces

Method:

1. Add balsamic vinegar, garlic, salt, and pepper in a bowl.
2. Marinate the mushrooms in it for at least an hour.
3. Heat a sauté pan. Add olive oil. When heated, add onions. Sauté for a couple of minutes.
4. Add the mushrooms along with the marinade. Cook for 7-8 minutes.
5. To serve, slit the burger buns. Place a lettuce leaf and a slice of tomato on one half of the bun. Place a mushroom and garlic. Cover with the other half of bun.
6. Serve with mustard and tomato ketchup or any other sauce of your choice. Suggested serving is avocado or roasted bell peppers.

Lentils with Mushrooms/Eggplant/Kale/Brussels sprouts:

Ingredients:

- 2 large Portobello mushrooms/eggplant/kale /Brussels sprouts, sliced
- 4.5 ounce lentils, cooked
- 2-3 tablespoons olive oil
- 1 tablespoon tomato paste
- 1 bunch flat leaf parsley, picked
- Sea salt to taste
- Pepper to taste
- Chilli flakes to taste

Method:

1. Heat a frying pan, add butter. Add mushroom or the vegetable you have used and sauté for 6-8 minutes until the mushrooms are tender.
2. Add lentils and tomato paste. Add salt, pepper and chilli flakes. Simmer for 5 minutes.
3. Serve hot garnished with parsley.

Lima Beans Hummus

Ingredients:

- ½ can lima beans
- 2 tablespoons lemon juice
- 1 clove garlic, minced
- ¼ teaspoon cumin, ground
- 2 tablespoons parsley, chopped
- ½ tablespoon paprika
- ¼ cup carrots, chopped
- ¼ cup celery, chopped
- Sea salt to taste.

Method:

1. Add to the blender lima beans, lemon juice, garlic, cumin and salt.
2. Blend until well pureed.
3. Transfer into a bowl. Add parsley and paprika. Mix well.
4. Refrigerate for a couple of hours.
5. Serve with carrots and celery.

Quinoa with nuts:

Ingredients:

- ½ cup quinoa (white or red)
- 1 cup water
- Fist full of goji berries
- Fist full of any nuts
- ½ teaspoon cumin seeds
- 1 tablespoon cilantro or fresh basil, chopped

Method:

1. Soak the quinoa in water for around 10 minutes
2. Strain the quinoa. Cook the quinoa with some water until soft.
3. Separately soak the goji berries in warm water for at least 10 minutes.
4. In a frying pan roast the cumin seeds. Add goji berries, nuts and quinoa.
5. Serve garnished with cilantro or parsley.

Brown Rice with Tomatoes:

Ingredients:

- ½ cup brown rice, cooked
- 7 cherry tomatoes
- ½ avocado
- 2 tablespoons cilantro, chopped
- 2 cloves garlic, minced
- ½ tablespoon olive oil
- Sea salt to taste
- Pepper powder to taste
- Chilli flakes to taste
- Any seasoning of your choice to taste
- Juice of ½ a lemon

Method:

1. Except brown rice, mix all the ingredients together.
2. Serve on a plate. Top with the mixed ingredients.
3. Adjust the seasonings to your taste.

Flax coated Chicken:

Ingredients:

- 2 chicken breasts, skinless, boneless
- 1 ½ tablespoons flax seeds, grounded
- ¼ cup almond meal
- ½ tablespoon extra virgin olive oil
- ½ tablespoon almond butter
- 1 tablespoon onions, finely chopped
- ½ teaspoon lemon juice
- ½ teaspoon sea salt or to taste
- ½ teaspoon parsley, chopped
- ½ teaspoon thyme, chopped
- ¼ teaspoon paprika
- Cayenne pepper to taste

Method:

1. Place the chicken breasts on a plastic wrap and pound it until the pieces are about ½ inch thick.
2. Mix together flax powder and almond meal.
3. In another bowl mix together the rest of the ingredients. Add the chicken pieces and coat well. Keep aside for ½ an hour to marinate.
4. Coat the chicken pieces with flax powder-almond meal mixture. Coat it well.
5. Place the chicken pieces on a baking dish. Place the dish on the top rack of the oven.
6. Bake in a preheated oven at 350 degrees for about 30 minutes or until done.

Pasta with Mushrooms and Brussels sprouts:

Ingredients:

- ½ pound whole wheat pasta (penne or rigatoni)
- 2 tablespoons olive oil
- ½ pound crimini mushrooms, sliced
- ½ pound Brussels sprouts, trimmed, shredded
- 2 cloves garlic, minced
- 1 teaspoon lemon zest, grated
- 2 tablespoons lemon juice
- Kosher salt to taste
- Freshly ground pepper to taste
- 1 small red bell pepper, cubed
- 1 small green pepper, cubed
- 1 small yellow bell pepper, cubed
- 1 teaspoon oregano, dried
- Red chilli flakes to taste

Method:

1. Cook pasta in a pot according to instructions. Strain and retain ¼ cup of the strained water. Transfer the pasta to the pot.
2. Meanwhile, heat a sauté pan. Add 1 tablespoon olive oil to it. When the oil is heated, add all the bell peppers, mushroom and a little of kosher salt. Sauté for 3-4 minutes.
3. Transfer the mushrooms with bell peppers into the pot.
4. Reheat the skillet. Add 1 tablespoon olive oil to it. Place on medium heat.
5. When oil is heated, add garlic, sauté for a few seconds. Add Brussels sprouts, salt and pepper. Sauté for about 5

minutes until the Brussels sprouts are soft. Add oregano and chilli flakes. Mix well and transfer into the pot. Now add the retained pasta water, lemon zest and lemon juice. Adjust the seasoning to your taste.

6. Serve hot.

Granola Parfait

Ingredients:

- 3 cups plain yogurt, unflavored and low fat
- 2 cups fruits, chopped or berries of your choice
- 3 tablespoons honey
- 1 cup rolled oats
- ½ cup nuts, chopped and seeds of your choice
- ½ tablespoon olive oil
- ½ teaspoon cinnamon
- ¼ teaspoon vanilla extract
- A pinch of salt

Method:

1. Chill the chopped fruits and yogurt.
2. In a large bowl mix together the oats, nuts, olive oil, cinnamon, vanilla, salt and ½ of the honey.
3. Spread evenly on a greased baking tray.
4. Bake in a preheated oven at 350 degrees F for around 45 minutes, stirring it every 15 minutes.
5. The granola should be golden brown if not then bake further for another 10-15 minutes Cool.
6. To serve, mix together the oats, and fruits. Add yogurt. Toss well.
7. Serve it in a glass. Top with remaining honey.

Black berry and blue berry delight:

Ingredients:

- 1/2 cup black berries
- ½ cup raspberries
- ½ tablespoon coconut oil
- 1 egg
- ½ cup coconut milk
- 2 tablespoons coconut nectar
- 1 ½ tablespoons coconut flour
- ¼ teaspoon vanilla extract
- ¼ teaspoon sea salt

Method:

1. Apply coconut oil at the bottom of a pie dish.
2. Add the raspberries and black berries to the dish.
3. Bake in a preheated oven at 400 degrees F for 5-7 minutes.
4. Whisk together the rest of the ingredients until a smooth batter is formed.
5. Pour this batter on the berries. Bake for 20-25 minutes or until firm.
6. Can serve hot or cold.

Almond muffins:

Ingredients:

- 1 ½ cups almond flour/meal
- 1 teaspoon baking powder
- 1 small zucchini , grated
- 5-6 black olives, pitted, roughly chopped
- ¼ cup coconut oil
- 1 tablespoon honey
- 1 tablespoon flax seeds, ground
- 1 teaspoon oregano, dried
- 1 teaspoon tarragon
- ¼ teaspoon sea salt

Method:

1. In a small bowl add flax seed powder and some warm water. Keep it aside for a few minutes.
2. Sift together almond flour, salt and baking powder.
3. In a large bowl add zucchini, olives, oil and honey. Mix well.
4. Add the almond flour mixture to this. Mix well.
5. Add oregano and tarragon. Mix well. Add the flax seed. Mix well. If the mixture is too thick, add some more oil.
6. Pour into greased muffin moulds.
7. Bake in a preheated oven at 375 degree F for about 30 minutes or until baked.
8. Remove from the moulds. Keep it in the refrigerator to set.
9. Ready   to   serve.

Berry pudding:

Ingredients:

- 2 tablespoons chia seeds
- ¾ glass coconut milk/almond milk
- ¼ teaspoon vanilla extract
- 1 tablespoon coconut butter or coconut oil (optional)
- Sea salt to taste
- 1 tablespoon honey
- ½ cup fresh raspberries/blue berries/black berries

Method:

1. Add chia seeds in warm coconut milk. Add coconut butter oil and salt. Mix well and keep aside for 15-20 minutes.
2. Add the raspberries and honey.
3. For variation, you can add banana or apple sauce instead of berries.
4. For variation, you can add cocoa powder to make chocolate pudding.

Chocolate muffins:

Ingredients:

- 1 cup teff flour
- ¼ cup rice flour
- ¼ cup corn meal flour
- ½ tablespoon baking powder
- ¼ teaspoon sea salt
- ¼ teaspoon nutmeg, grounded
- ¼ teaspoon chilli powder
- ¼ cup cocoa powder
- 1 drop culinary lavender oil
- 1 tablespoon flaxseed powdered
- 1 ½ tablespoon warm water
- ¼ cup honey (add more if you like it sweeter)
- ¼ cup almond milk
- ¼ cup coconut oil
- ¼ cup olive oil
- 6 tablespoons dark chocolate (70%), chopped finely

Method:

1. In a small bowl add flaxseed powder and water and keep aside for 15-20 minutes.
2. In another bowl add coconut milk, honey, almond milk and culinary lavender oil.
3. Mix well. Add the dry ingredients to this. Also add the flax seeds. Mix well to form a batter. If the batter is too thick add some more almond milk.
4. Add chocolate pieces. Stir well.
5. Pour into greased muffin moulds.

6. Bake in a preheated oven at 375 degrees for 25-30 minutes or until baked well.

7. When warm, remove from mould.

Conclusion

Thank you again for downloading this book!

I hope this book was able to help you to know more about hypothyroidism and how to treat it with the right foods and other natural means.

The next step is simply to put into action what you have read in this book and hopefully see great results soon. Share it with friends so they too can benefit from the helpful knowledge in this book. Even if they don't have hypothyroidism, it pays to know how to avoid getting the illness.

Finally, if you enjoyed this book, please take the time to share your thoughts and post a review on Amazon. It'd be greatly appreciated!

The Following Is A Sample From The Author's Book – The Autoimmune Menu: Eating Well With Autoimmune Ailments

http://www.amazon.com/dp/B00EYRBVQW

Chapter 2

Diet Considerations

Choosing the right food items for the recipes may be a bit confusing at first. However, people with **autoimmune disease** can make the most out of their diet by making sure that they know some of the guidelines that can help them effectively design their personalized diet programs. This part of the book will tell you some of the considerations that you have to make when preparing the recipes that can help manage some of the symptoms that the autoimmune diseases can bring.

Gluten

When it comes to the gluten based autoimmune disorders, you have to get rid of the food items that contain gluten. You should do this for the rest of your life. Recent studies have shown that the bacterial components in your stomach may be considered as one of the probable environmental factors that can cause digestive system based autoimmune disorders. One of the most common disorders under this category is the celiac disease. Although the experts need to conduct more research regarding this field, it is an established fact that if the people with the condition are diagnosed early in the phase and can readily comply with the recommended gluten free diet, the risk of acquiring complications from the diet may be significantly lowered. Some of the complications that the diet can prevent are gastrointestinal cancer and osteoporosis.

Going for food items that do not contain gluten may be considered as a famous regimen for most of the autoimmune disorders out there. Aside from celiac disease, this diet pointer may also apply for people with multiple sclerosis, systemic lupus erythematosus, and rheumatoid arthritis. In this regard, you should keep in mind that the recent studies have not yet proven that the gluten free diet approach can address the rest of the disorders with autoimmune characteristics. One way to tell if this is appropriate for you is to undergo the gluten sensitivity test.

Oxidation

One of the most promising dietary approaches that the dieticians are rooting for is the antioxidant and anti-inflammatory diet approach. According to these experts, the approach can help provide equilibrium for the immune system of the person with the condition. On top of that, this dietary approach can aid in significantly reducing the amount of oxidative stress that the body systems of the person with the condition is currently going through. This is important because the heightened immune system response can aid in elevating the levels of free radicals in the body. In turn, this can contribute in speeding up the deterioration for most of the body systems of the person with the autoimmune disorder.

Omega-3 Fatty Acids

The probable benefits of the omega 3 fatty acids in addressing the **autoimmune disease** have fascinated the experts for the longest time. This acid group contains powerful immunomodulatory potentials. This is especially true for the fish oil. The anti-inflammatory effects of omega-3 fatty acids may make them helpful in managing the symptoms brought about by these disorders. At present, the experts were able to harbor positive results after incorporating this nutrient in the diet programs for people with the following disorders: (1) rheumatoid arthritis; (2) multiple sclerosis; (3) systemic lupus erythematosus; and (4) Crohn's disease. Most of the high level studies in the research field came up with the assumption that the omega-3 fatty acids can help in significantly reducing the presence of tender points in some autoimmune disorders. Also, these studies stated that the need for the use of nonsteroidal anti-inflammatory drugs has been drastically reduced since the omega-3 fatty acids have been incorporated in the participants' diet programs.

Chapter 3

Food Group Choices

The autoimmune disorders are considered as serious and painful conditions where the immune system of the body mistakenly identifies the natural occurring cells as foreign ones. As a result, they tend to attack these harmless cells. This part of the book will discuss some of the specific food groups that you may incorporate in your diet program. Numerous studies have already proven that these food groups can help address the symptoms for people with **autoimmune disease**. As much as possible, you must include the following food groups in your diet to make sure that the symptoms of the autoimmune disorders will be well managed.

Whole Grain
Just as you should avoid additives such as shortenings and processed fats, you should also avoid the processed carbohydrates. Instead of going for the processed flour, processed sugar, and the refined ones, you have to make sure that you will select the whole grain counterparts. As much as possible, you have to make sure that you will choose the fresh

bread that has been locally produced over the conventional bread loaves that you can readily purchase in your local grocery store. Also, you have to go for the natural sources of sugar instead of the refined ones. In this regard, you may choose from the following sweet additions: (1) honey; (2) molasses; and (3) maple syrup.

Vegetables

Even if it is considered a given fact, you should not stray away from the use of fresh vegetables to help you spice up your dishes. Actually, you can consider any type of fresh vegetable as a good choice that you can readily include in your special diet if ever you are suffering from an autoimmune disorder. It is definitely crucial to keep your diet well balanced by incorporating whole food items like this in your diet. This means that as much as possible, you have to stay away from the processed counterparts that you may find in your store. In effect, these food items can help make sure that your body will be operating in the best way possible. This is especially important during the exacerbation phases of your autoimmune disorder. In this regard, you have to capitalize mostly on organic vegetables because they tend to have higher concentrations of nutrients in them compared to the processed ones.

Dairy

Another ideal food choice is the dairy. However, you have to make sure that you will opt for the easy to digest varieties to help you prevent stress for your digestive system. Some of the dairy based food items that you can incorporate in your diet program are yogurt and eggs. Also, you have to choose the low fat versions to help you get rid of the chance for the **autoimmune disease** to develop over time.

Olive Oil

Most of the people know that incorporating the extra virgin olive oil in your diet can help in alleviating the signs and symptoms of autoimmune diseases. Typically, the extra virgin olive oil is used as the main cooking ingredient. Compared to the conventional cooking oil that healthy people incorporate in their dishes, the extra virgin olive oil is important for the treatment of the symptoms because the digestive system can easily process and absorb the nutrients so your body can use up the rest of the components for continuous functions. When this happens smoothly, you can rest assured that your body will not likely have to deal with a lot of potential stress triggers that can eventually start an episode of exacerbation. Aside from fried foods, you may also use this type of oil for baking.

Chapter 4

Protein Dishes

In this chapter, you will discover some of the protein based recipes that you can definitely include in your daily diet program. Protein is important because for people with autoimmune disorder because they can help in the development of your major muscle groups. Aside from that, this nutrient can also contribute in the production of the reinforcement that the body will use for physical recovery. This is especially important during events such as wound healing and the various inflammation processes. Included in this part are some of the protein rich recipes that can tickle your taste buds. These are all easy to create.

Baked Beef Brisket

Among the most common protein sources that you can count on, beef may be considered as one of the staples for your **autoimmune disease** diet program. In this light, you may cook up baked beef brisket as your next beef dish. This recipe goes well with the sweet potatoes. For this recipe, you need to prepare the following:

- Two teaspoons of scallion salt or onion powder
- One teaspoon of coriander
- Three tablespoons of white peppercorns or whole black ones
- One to 1.5 teaspoons of smoked Hungarian variety paprika
- One teaspoon of thyme
- Three to four pounds of corned beef brisket (preferably with fat)

Initially, you have to preheat your oven to 275 degrees Celsius. Next, you need to line the dish with aluminum foil. You have to make sure that the dish is large enough for your meat to expand. You have to place another layer of heavy duty foil over the first layer. After this, you may set up the meat with the skin against the surface of the aluminum foil. For the seasoning, you have to thoroughly combine all the spices that you have initially prepared and rub them on top of the beef. After this, you may loosely wrap the foil on the meat. You have to bake the beef in the over for two hours. After taking out the beef from the oven and uncovering the meat, you may then turn it over such that the fat side is up. You can tightly wrap the meat in the foil once more as soon as the juice flowed out. At this point, you need to place the meat in the over for another one to two hours.

http://www.amazon.com/dp/B00EYRBVQW

www.ingramcontent.com/pod-product-compliance
Lightning Source LLC
Chambersburg PA
CBHW071237280526
45787CB00002B/968